What We Want Our Friends and Family to Know about Parkinson's

Eugenia H. Parker

and

Friends

DEDICATION

This is dedicated to our friends and family who have helped us as we have dealt with the effects of Parkinson's. And also to the people with Parkinson's who feel others don't understand their issues.

I would also dedicate this to my Mother, Betty and my Daughter, Elizabeth who have always believed I could do anything and to David who has encouraged me and helped me in a million ways.

CONTENTS

ACKNOWLEDGMENTS

Most people in our class have provided various issues and suggestions for the book. The class members involved in the creation reviewed the pages as they were constructed and helped determine how to phrase issues. This was a group effort of the following people: Mia Reager, Marianne Guffanti, Teeter Harte, Frank Gemmato, Bree Moore, Richard Lindstrom, Mark McGranaghan, Sheldon Hill, Lulu Mosman, Linda Bradley, Tony Vaughn, JoAnne Hall, Randy Craig, Neil Arden and others.

We attend an exercise class that specializes in helping Parkinson's patients. Most, but not all, of us have Parkinson's. The class is under the direction of our dedicated teacher, Breanna Moore.

We first want to thank all our friends and families for their help and understanding. Sometimes we don't like to make suggestions because we know you do so much for us already. We hope this little book will help your interactions with people with Parkinson's disease, PD.

To those with PD, we say keep moving as long as you can and in whatever manner you can. It really makes a difference.

This book is designed so you can individualize it to the issues you have, because all Parkinson's patients are different. There are spaces to write the specific ways to help you. There are blank pages, tabs and sample pages in the back of the book.

Thank you for caring

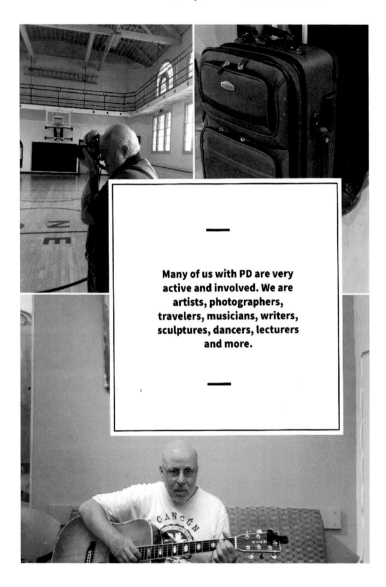

Many of us with PD are very active and involved. We are artists, photographers, travelers, musicians, writers, sculptures, dancers, lecturers and more.

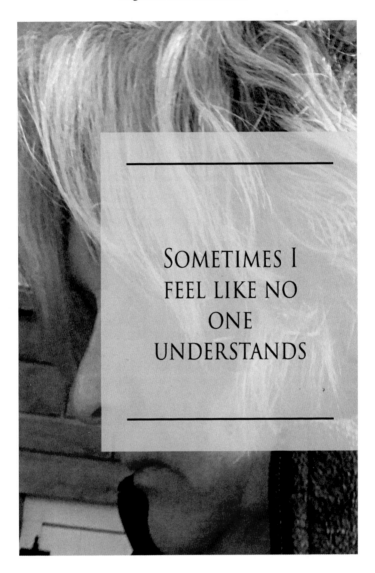

SOMETIMES I
FEEL LIKE NO
ONE
UNDERSTANDS

PD IS A DISEASE OF THE BRAIN WHICH CAUSES VARIOUS SYMPTOMS. PLEASE TRY NOT TO COMPARE MY SYMPTOMS WITH OTHERS WHO HAVE THE DISEASE. IT AFFECTS EVERYONE IN A DIFFERENT WAY.

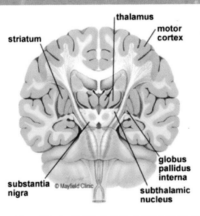

Figure 2. A cross section of the brain. The impulse for body movement begins in the motor cortex of the brain. The basal ganglia are responsible for activating and inhibiting specific circuits or feedback loops.

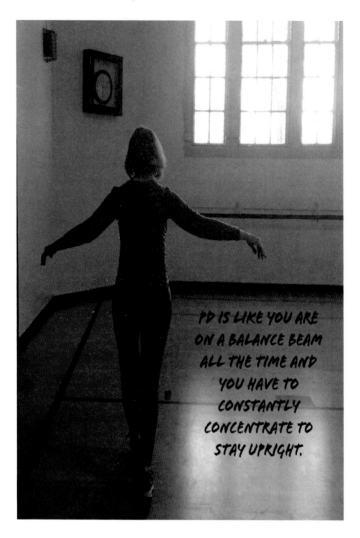

PD IS LIKE YOU ARE
ON A BALANCE BEAM
ALL THE TIME AND
YOU HAVE TO
CONSTANTLY
CONCENTRATE TO
STAY UPRIGHT.

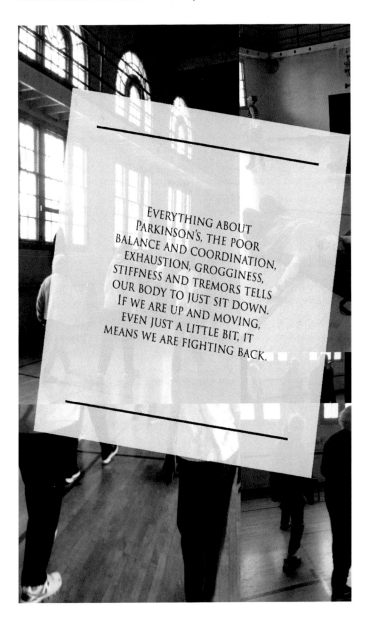

EVERYTHING ABOUT PARKINSON'S, THE POOR BALANCE AND COORDINATION, EXHAUSTION, GROGGINESS, STIFFNESS AND TREMORS TELLS OUR BODY TO JUST SIT DOWN. IF WE ARE UP AND MOVING, EVEN JUST A LITTLE BIT, IT MEANS WE ARE FIGHTING BACK.

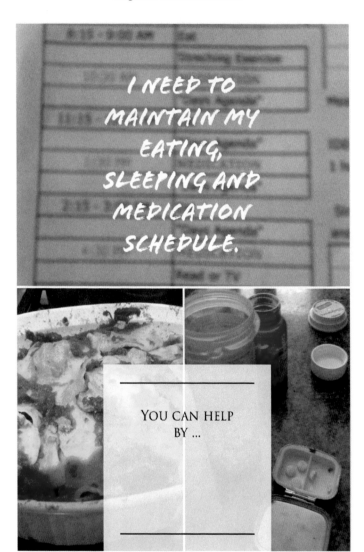

I NEED TO MAINTAIN MY EATING, SLEEPING AND MEDICATION SCHEDULE.

YOU CAN HELP BY ...

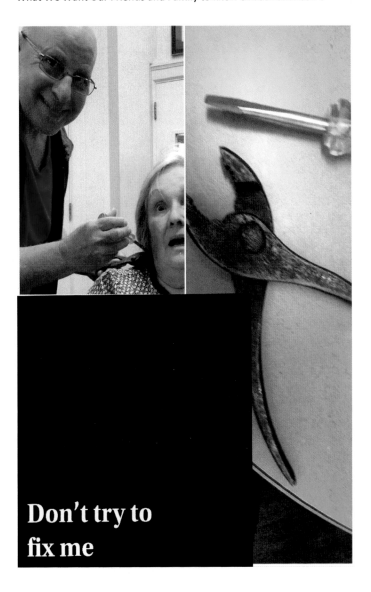

Don't try to fix me

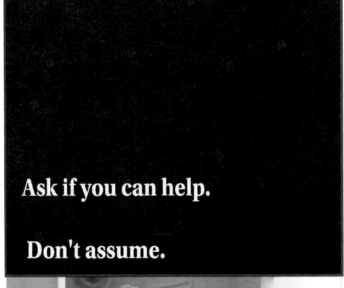

Ask if you can help.

Don't assume.

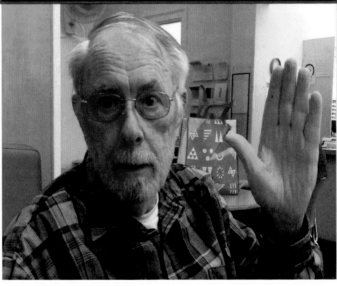

If I need help putting on my jacket I'll ask for it. Otherwise please let me do it my way,unusual though it may appear.

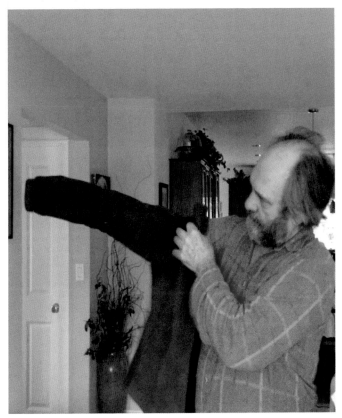

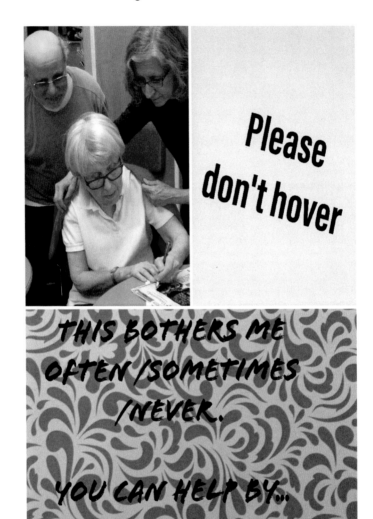

I have good days and bad days.

Mon	Tue	Wed	Thr	Fri	Sat	Sun
			1	2	3	4
5	6	7	8	9	10	11
12	13	14	15	16	17	18
19	20	21	22	23	24	25
26	27	28	29	30		

19

Sometimes it's difficult to start a task. It's called ' The Initial Response'.

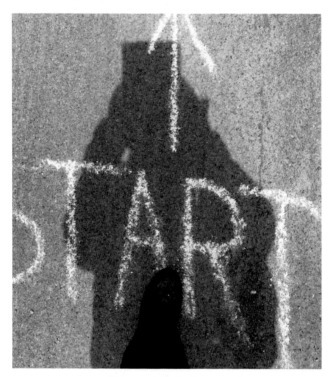

You can help by ...

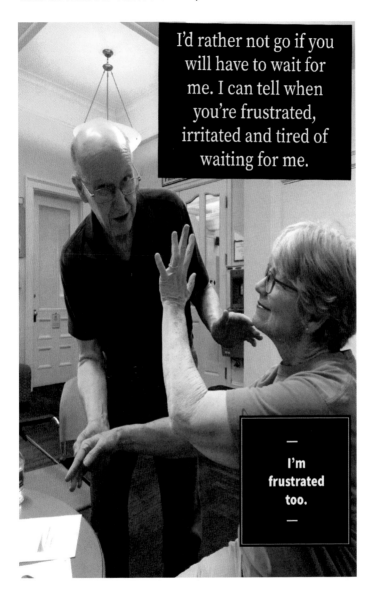

I'd rather not go if you will have to wait for me. I can tell when you're frustrated, irritated and tired of waiting for me.

—
I'm frustrated too.
—

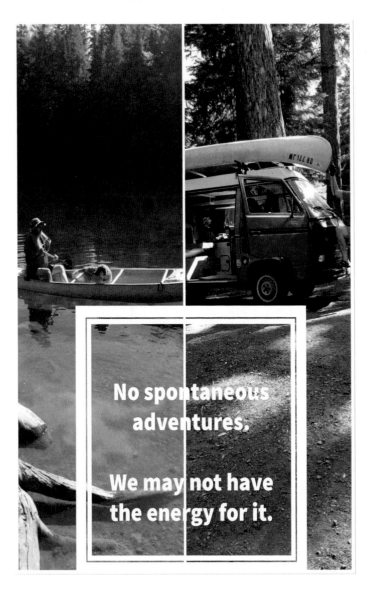

No spontaneous
adventures.

We may not have
the energy for it.

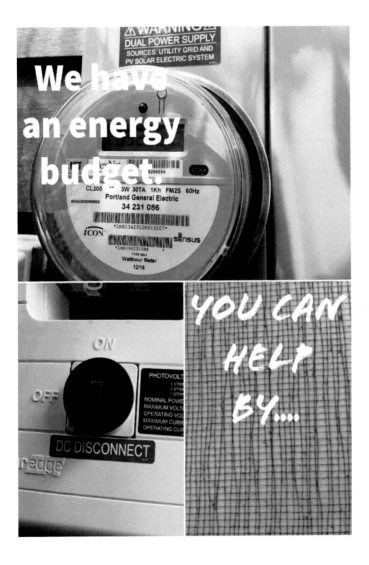

SOMETIMES I DON'T WANT TO GO SOMEPLACE OR DO SOMETHING BECAUSE IT TAKES MORE EFFORT THAN I HAVE.

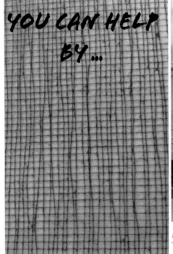

YOU CAN HELP BY...

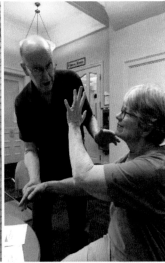

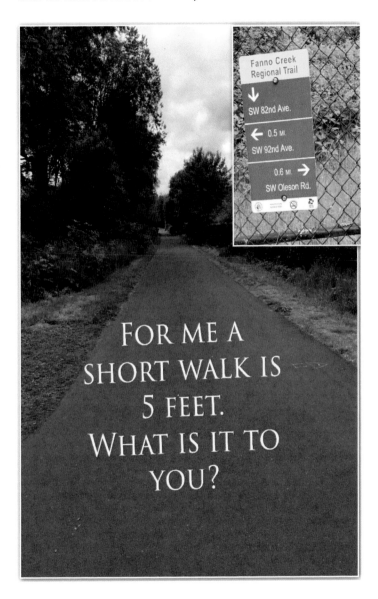

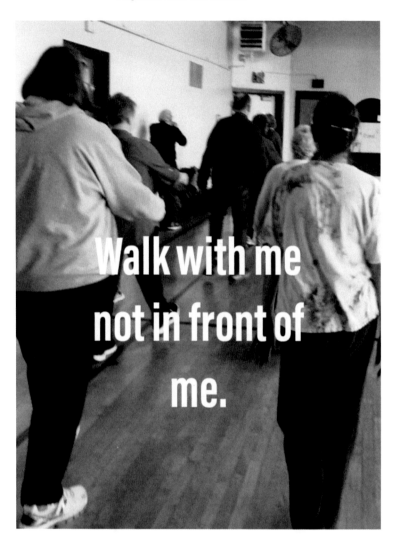

Walk with me not in front of me.

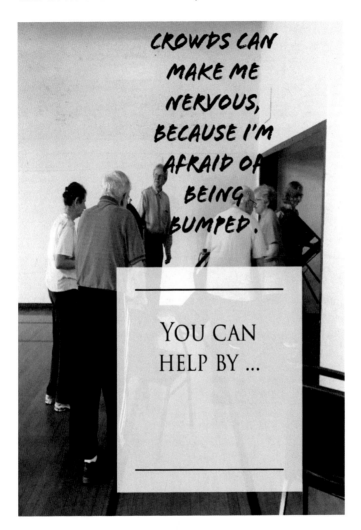

CROWDS CAN MAKE ME NERVOUS, BECAUSE I'M AFRAID OF BEING BUMPED.

YOU CAN HELP BY ...

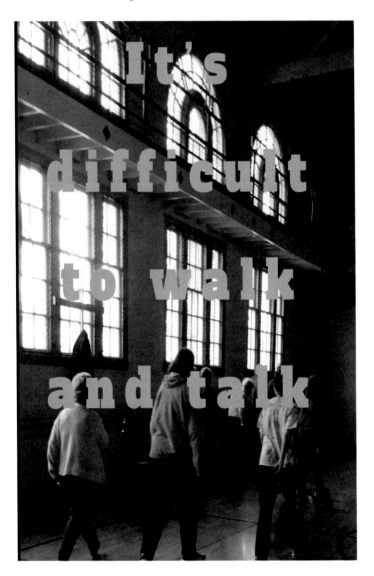

It's difficult to walk and talk

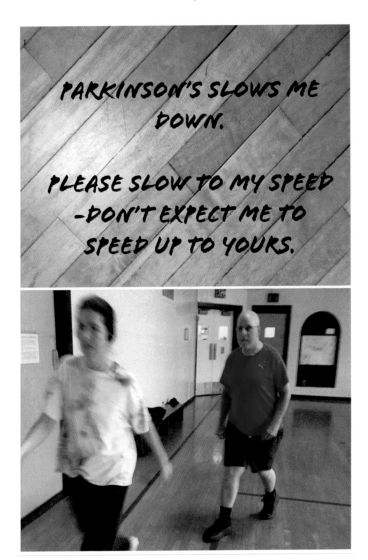

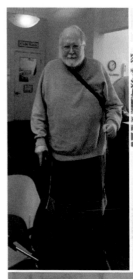

SOMETIMES I CAN'T MOVE AND I APPEAR FROZEN. IT'S UNPREDICTABLE AND TEMPORARY. I KNOW SOME TRICKS. I'LL THAW OUT IN A MINUTE AND BE ABLE TO MOVE.

I DO / DON'T EXPERIENCE THIS.
YOU CAN HELP BY ...

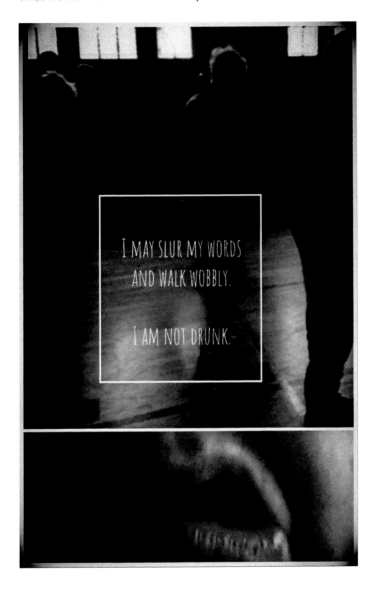

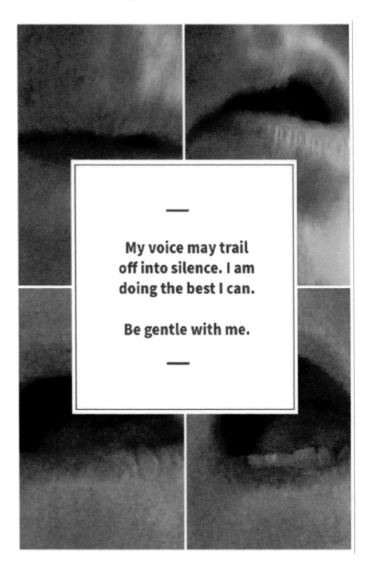

—

My voice may trail
off into silence. I am
doing the best I can.

Be gentle with me.

—

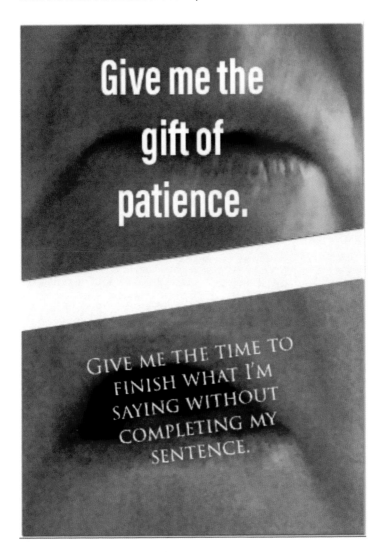

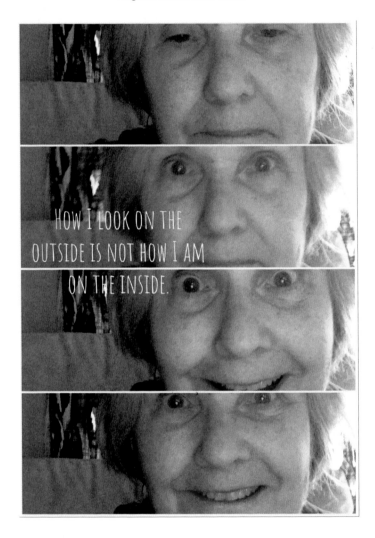

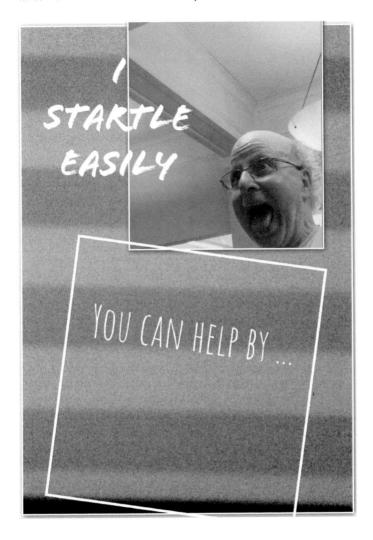

I may get angry quickly

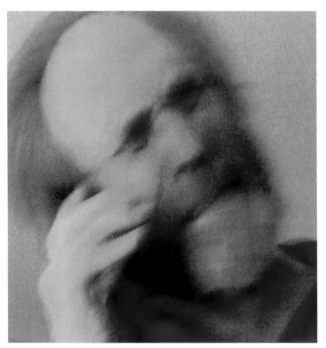

I do this sometimes/never/often
you can help by...

SOMETIMES I
PANIC AND IT
LOOKS LIKE
AGGRESSION.

_____

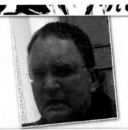

I do / do not
experience this.
You can help by

.....

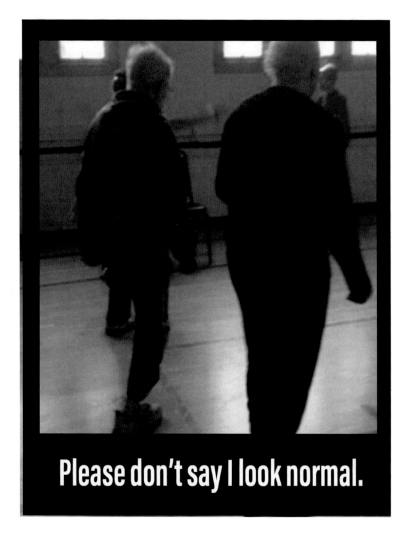

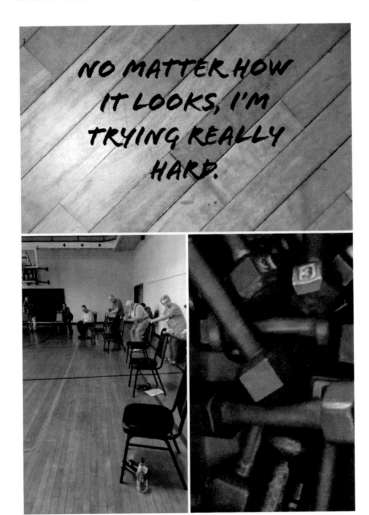

NO MATTER HOW IT LOOKS, I'M TRYING REALLY HARD.

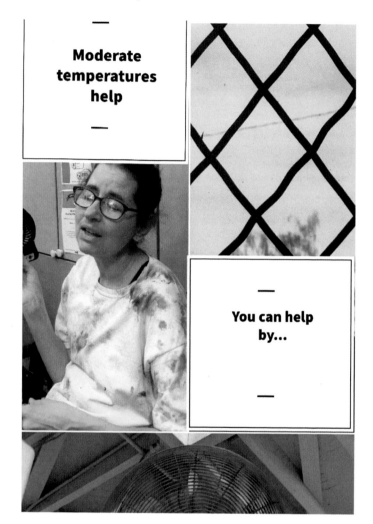

Moderate temperatures help

You can help by...

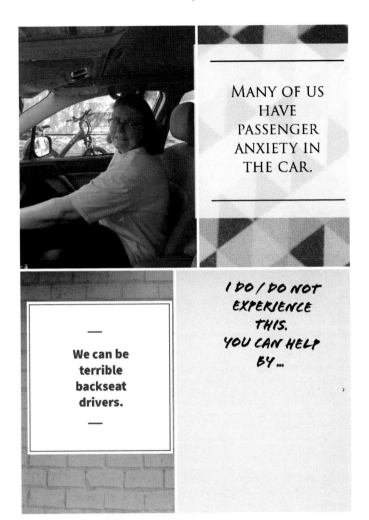

MANY OF US HAVE PASSENGER ANXIETY IN THE CAR.

We can be terrible backseat drivers.

I DO / DO NOT EXPERIENCE THIS. YOU CAN HELP BY ...

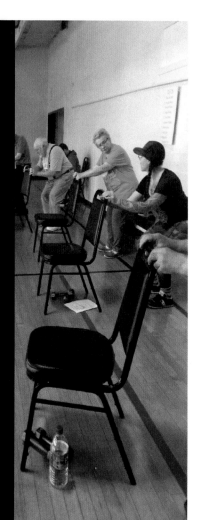

A lot of effort goes into just living.

Trying to stand up
straight
Trying to keep
moving
Trying to
participate
Trying to quiet the
anxiety
Trying not to give
up

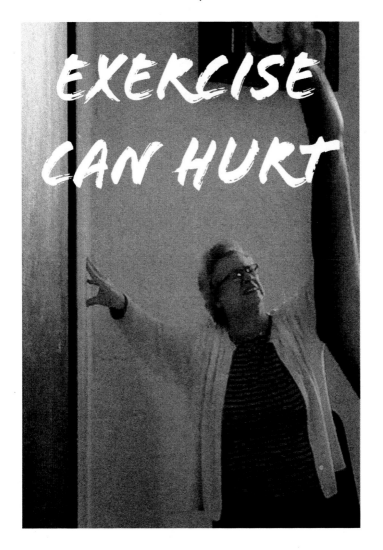

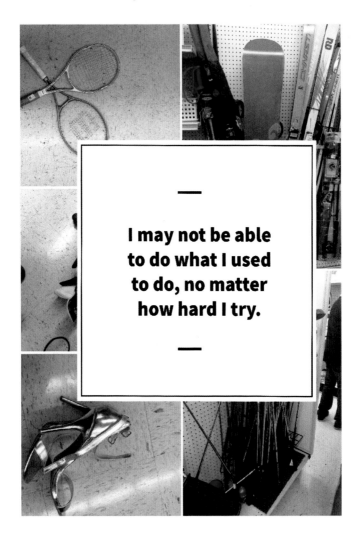

—

I may not be able
to do what I used
to do, no matter
how hard I try.

—

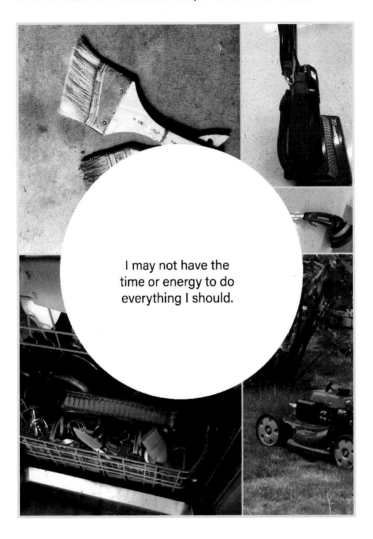

I may not have the time or energy to do everything I should.

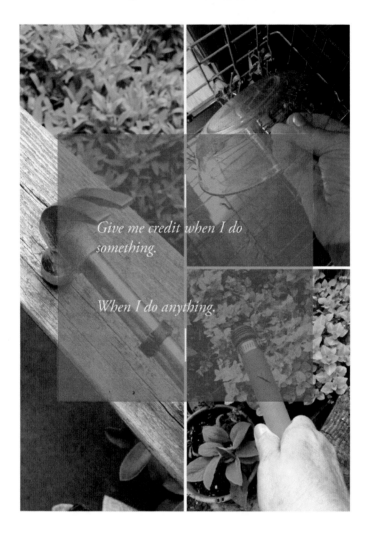

Give me credit when I do something.

When I do anything.

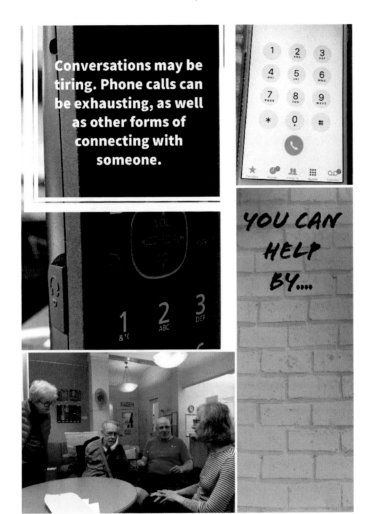

Conversations may be tiring. Phone calls can be exhausting, as well as other forms of connecting with someone.

YOU CAN HELP BY....

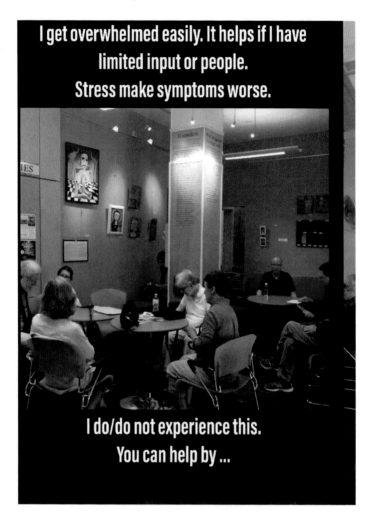

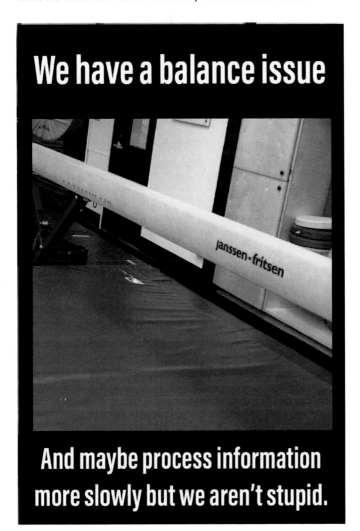

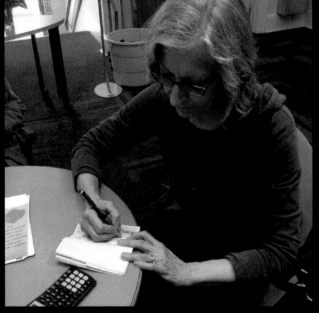

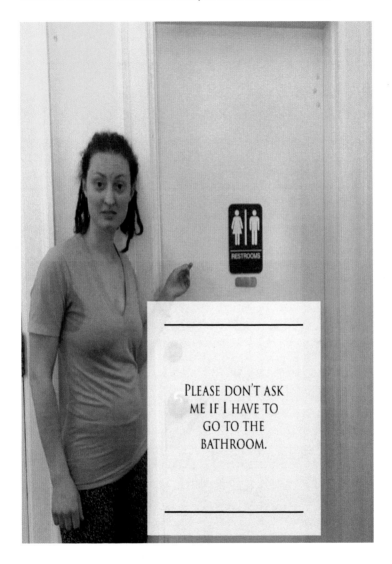

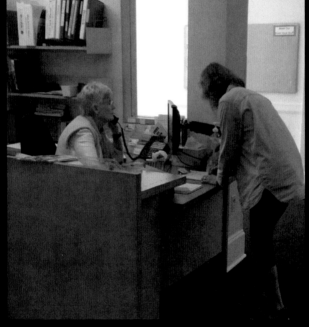

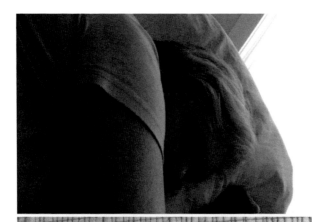

SOME OF US DON'T JUST WANT TO TAKE A NAP, WE HAVE TO TAKE A NAP. SLEEP IS A WAY OF RECHARGING OUR BATTERY AND HELPS US MAKE IT THROUGH THE AFTERNOON.

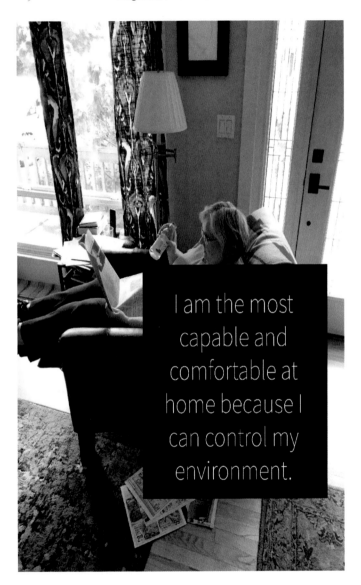

I am the most capable and comfortable at home because I can control my environment.

Talking about the future is difficult.

Please wait for us to bring it up.

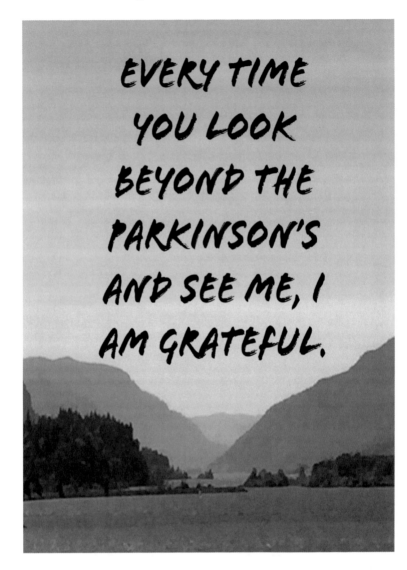

EVERY TIME YOU LOOK BEYOND THE PARKINSON'S AND SEE ME, I AM GRATEFUL.

Please help me with the following symptoms:

Please help me deal with the following issues:

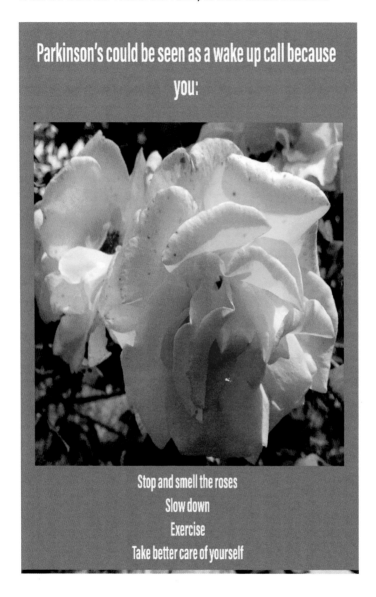

Parkinson's could be seen as a wake up call because you:

Stop and smell the roses
Slow down
Exercise
Take better care of yourself

THIS IS AN EXAMPLE OF HOW THE PAGES CAN BE PERSONALIZED

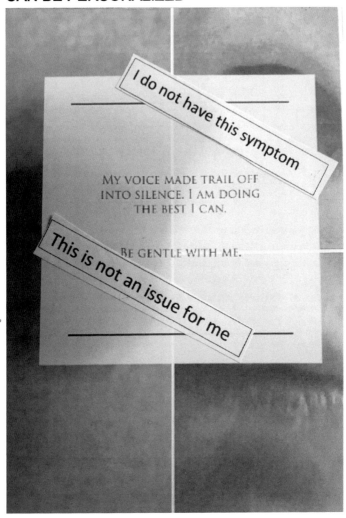

THIS IS AN EXAMPLE OF HOW THE PAGES CAN BE PERSONALIZED

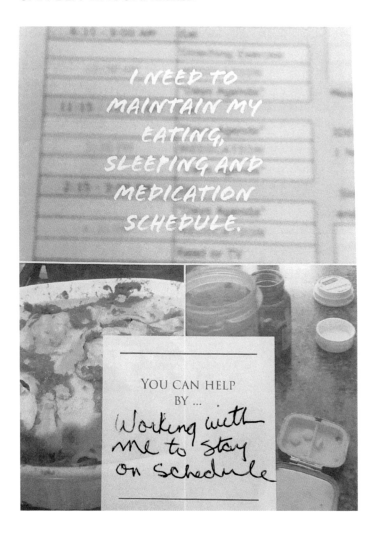

Tabs that can be cut out and pasted on pages that do not apply to you

I do not have this symptom

I do not have this symptom

I do not have this symptom

I do not have this symptom

I do not have this symptom

I do not have this symptom

I do not have this symptom

Tabs that can be cut out and pasted on pages that do not apply to you

This is not an issue for me

This is not an issue for me

This is not an issue for me

This is not an issue for me

This is not an issue for me

This is not an issue for me

Eugenia Parker and Friends

Made in the USA
Las Vegas, NV
10 December 2020

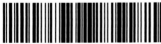